MW01127417

Dash Diet Cookbook for Beginners

Stay Fit, Lose Weight With Delicious, Easy-To-Make Recipes for a Healthy Lifestyle

Winifred Clark

TABLE OF CONTENTS

INTRODUCTION

Many people who follow the DASH diet have lost weight due to healthy eating choices. Healthy food choices can help you lose weight, but ultimately the "DASH diet" will help you make these choices for the rest of your life.

If you want to lose unwanted pounds, we recommend a diet program or diet product that is conducive to your lifestyle and weight loss goals, easy to follow and apply everywhere.

DASH Diet for Weight Loss uses proven techniques to help you change your eating habits and follow the Dash diet. This diet is not focused on weight loss, but when coupled with exercise, their list of recommended healthy foods can still help you lose weight. So you learn how to start the diet and how to behave in phase 1. If you want to get a little closer to the "DASH diet," you can also use the menu when shopping and use it as a cookbook when shopping.

In addition to eating foods for low blood pressure, the DASH diet can also lower LDL cholesterol and help you lose weight if you are overweight or obese.

In addition, increasing your fruit and vegetable intake and focusing on whole grains helps you feel full the longer you eat, and can help you eat less to avoid weight loss. Finally, there are many other benefits of the DASH diet that can be maintained in the long term. You can include small amounts of high-density foods and have what you don't need to lose weight. Some foods are not included in their scope, such as fruits, vegetables, nuts, seeds and legumes, but some may be included.

Because the DASH diet eliminates or promotes certain food groups, people with dietary restrictions can follow them without restriction. Give up sweets altogether by following the DASH diet or simply by forgoing them and eating fruits, vegetables, nuts, seeds and legumes.

Although the DASH diet is not designed to lose weight, following these guidelines can help you eat healthier and avoid junk, which often means lower numbers on the scales. Whether you like the "DASH" diet or hope to lose weight in the long term, you need a program like Noom to help you tackle it in the most balanced way. The tips, tricks and techniques we've shared over the years # offer all the skills you need to stay at Dash Diet for weight loss.

If you are used to eating many ready meals and fast food, you may want to gradually switch to the DASH diet. Start with more vegetables, switch to low-fat dairy products or reduce meat consumption. If you follow this diet, you will eat less junk food and more fruit and vegetables and less meat and dairy products.

BREAKFAST

1. Mediterranean Toast

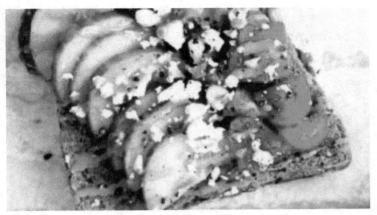

Preparation time: 10 minutes

Cooking time: 0 minutes

Servings: 2

Ingredients:

- 1 ½ tsp. reduced-Fat crumbled feta
- 3 sliced Greek olives
- ¼ mashed avocado
- 1 slice good whole wheat bread
- 1 tbsp. roasted red pepper hummus
- 3 sliced cherry tomatoes
- 1 sliced hardboiled egg

Directions:

1. First, toast the bread and top it with ¼ mashed avocado and 1 tablespoon hummus. Add the cherry tomatoes, olives, hardboiled egg, and feta. To taste, season with salt and pepper.

Nutrition: Calories: 333.7, Fat: 17 g, Carbs: 33.3 g, Protein: 16.3 g, Sugars: 1 g, Sodium: 19 mg

2. Instant Banana Oatmeal

Preparation time: 1 minute

Cooking time: 2 minutes

Servings: 1

Ingredients:

- 1 mashed ripe banana
- ½ c. water
- ½ c. quick oats

Directions:

1. Measure the oats and water into a microwave-safe bowl and stir to combine. Place bowl in microwave and heat on high for 2 minutes. Remove the bowl, then stir in the mashed banana and serve.

Nutrition: Calories: 243, Fat: 3 g, Carbs: 50 g, Protein: 6 g, Sugars: 20 g, Sodium: 30 mg

3. Almond Butter-Banana Smoothie

Preparation time: 5 minutes

Cooking time: 0 minutes

Servings: 1

Ingredients:

- 1 tbsp. Almond butter
- ½ c. ice cubes
- ½ c. packed spinach
- 1 peeled and a frozen medium banana
- 1 c. Fat-free milk

Directions:

1. Blend all the listed fixing above in a powerful blender until smooth and creamy. Serve and enjoy.

Nutrition: Calories: 293, Fat: 9.8 g, Carbs: 42.5 g, Protein: 13.5 g, Sugars: 12 g, Sodium: 40 mg

4. Brown Sugar Cinnamon Oatmeal

Preparation time: 1 minute

Cooking time: 3 minutes

Servings: 4

Ingredients:

- ½ tsp. ground cinnamon
- 1 ½ tsp. pure vanilla extract
- ¼ c. light brown sugar
- 2 c. low- Fat milk
- 1 1/3 c. quick oats

Directions:

1. Put the milk plus vanilla into a medium saucepan and boil over medium-high heat.

2. Lower the heat to medium once it boils. Mix in oats, brown sugar, plus cinnamon, and cook, stirring2–3 minutes. Serve immediately.

Nutrition: Calories: 208, Fat: 3 g, Carbs: 38 g, Protein: 8 g, Sugars: 15 g, Sodium: 33 mg

5. Buckwheat Pancakes with Vanilla Almond Milk

Preparation time: 10 minutes

Cooking time: 10 minutes

Servings: 1

Ingredients:

- ½ c. unsweetened vanilla almond milk
- 2-4 packets natural sweetener
- 1/8 tsp. salt
- ½ cup buckwheat flour
- ½ tsp. double-acting baking powder

Directions:

1. Prepare a nonstick pancake griddle and spray with the cooking spray, place over medium heat. Whisk the buckwheat flour, salt, baking powder, and stevia in a small bowl and stir in the almond milk after.

2. Onto the pan, scoop a large spoonful of batter, cook until bubbles no longer pop on the surface and the entire surface looks dry and (2-4 minutes). Flip and cook for another 2-4 minutes. Repeat with all the remaining batter.

Nutrition: Calories: 240, Fat: 4.5 g, Carbs: 2 g, Protein: 11 g, Sugars: 17 g, Sodium: 38 mg

LUNCH

6. Secret Asian Green Beans

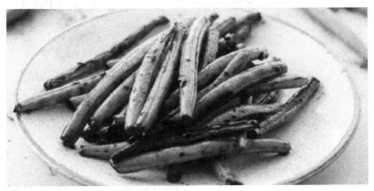

Preparation time: 10 minutes

Cooking time: 2 hours

Servings: 10

Ingredients:

- 16 cups green beans, halved
- 3 tablespoons olive oil
- ¼ cup tomato sauce, salt-free
- ½ cup coconut sugar
- ¾ teaspoon low sodium soy sauce
- Pinch of pepper

Directions:

1. Add green beans, coconut sugar, pepper tomato sauce, soy sauce, and oil to your Slow Cooker.

2. Stir well.

3. Place lid and cook on LOW for 3 hours.

4. Divide between serving platters and serve.

5. Enjoy!

Nutrition: Calories: 200; Fat: 4g; Carbohydrates: 12g; Protein: 3g

7. Excellent Acorn Mix

Preparation time: 10 minutes

Cooking time: 7 hours

Servings: 10

Ingredients:

- 2 acorn squash, peeled and cut into wedges
- 16 ounces cranberry sauce, unsweetened
- ¼ teaspoon cinnamon powder
- Pepper to taste

Directions:

1. Add acorn wedges to your Slow Cooker.
2. Add cranberry sauce, cinnamon, raisins and pepper.
3. Stir.
4. Place lid and cook on LOW for 7 hours.
5. Serve and enjoy!

Nutrition: Calories: 200; Fat: 3g; Carbohydrates: 15g; Protein: 2g

8. Crunchy Almond Chocolate Bars

Preparation time: 10 minutes

Cooking time: 2 hours and 30 minutes

Servings: 12

Ingredients:

- 1 egg white
- ¼ cup coconut oil, melted
- 1 cup coconut sugar
- ½ teaspoon vanilla extract
- 1 teaspoon baking powder
- 1 ½ cups almond meal
- ½ cup dark chocolate chips

Directions:

1. Take a bowl and add sugar, oil, vanilla extract, egg white, almond flour, baking powder and mix it well.
2. Fold in chocolate chips and stir.
3. Line Slow Cooker with parchment paper.
4. Grease.
5. Add the cookie mix and press on bottom.
6. Place lid and cook on LOW for 2 hours 30 minutes.
7. Take cookie sheet out and let it cool.
8. Cut in bars and enjoy!

Nutrition: Calories: 200; Fat: 2g; Carbohydrates: 13g; Protein: 6g

9. Lettuce and Chicken Platter

Preparation time: 10 minutes

Cooking time: 20 minutes

Servings: 6

Ingredients:

- 2 cups chicken, cooked and coarsely chopped
- ½ head ice berg lettuce, sliced and chopped
- 1 celery rib, chopped
- 1 medium apple, cut
- ½ red bell pepper, deseeded and chopped
- 6-7 green olives, pitted and halved
- 1 red onion, chopped
- For dressing
- 1 tablespoon raw honey
- 2 tablespoons lemon juice
- Salt and pepper to taste

Directions:

1. Cut the vegetables and transfer them to your Salad Bowl.
2. Add olives.
3. Chop the cooked chicken and transfer to your Salad bowl.

4. Prepare dressing by mixing the ingredients listed under Dressing.

5. Pour the dressing into the Salad bowl.

6. Toss and enjoy!

Nutrition: Calories: 296; Fat: 21g; Carbohydrates: 9g; Protein: 18g

10. Greek Lemon Chicken Bowl

Preparation time: 10 minutes

Cooking time: 15 minutes

Servings: 6

Ingredients:

- 2 cups chicken, cooked and chopped
- 2 cans chicken broth, fat free
- 2 medium carrots, chopped
- ¼ teaspoon pepper
- 2 tablespoons parsley, snipped
- ¼ cup lemon juice
- 1 can cream chicken soup, fat free, low sodium
- ½ cup onion, chopped
- 1 garlic clove, minced

Directions:

1. Take a pot and add all the ingredients except parsley into it.
2. Season with salt and pepper.
3. Bring the mix to a boil over medium-high heat.
4. Reduce the heat and simmer for 15 minutes.
5. Garnish with parsley.
6. Serve hot and enjoy!

Nutrition: Calories: 520; Fat: 33g; Carbohydrates: 31g; Protein: 30g

DINNER

11. Amazing Sesame Breadsticks

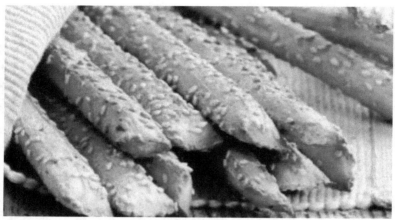

Preparation time: 10 minutes

Cooking time: 20 minutes

Servings: 5

Ingredients:

- 1 egg white
- 2 tablespoons almond flour
- 1 teaspoon Himalayan pink sunflower seeds
- 1 tablespoon extra-virgin olive oil
- ½ teaspoon sesame seeds

Directions:

1. Pre-heat your oven to 320 degrees F.

2. Line a baking sheet with parchment paper and keep it on the side.

3. Take a bowl and whisk in egg whites, add flour and half of sunflower seeds and olive oil.

4. Knead until you have a smooth dough.

5. Divide into 4 pieces and roll into breadsticks.

6. Place on prepared sheet and brush with olive oil, sprinkle sesame seeds and remaining sunflower seeds.

7. Bake for 20 minutes.

8. Serve and enjoy!

Nutrition: Total Carbs: 1.1g; Fiber: 1g; Protein: 1.6g; Fat: 5g

12. Brown Butter Duck Breast

Preparation time: 5 minutes

Cooking time: 25 minutes

Servings: 3

Ingredients:

- 1 whole 6 ounce duck breast, skin on
- Pepper to taste
- 1 head radicchio, 4 ounces, core removed
- ¼ cup unsalted butter
- 6 fresh sage leaves, sliced

Directions:

1. Pre-heat your oven to 400 degree F.
2. Pat duck breast dry with paper towel.
3. Season with pepper.
4. Place duck breast in skillet and place it over medium heat, sear for 3-4 minutes each side.
5. Turn breast over and transfer skillet to oven.
6. Roast for 10 minutes (uncovered).
7. Cut radicchio in half.
8. Remove and discard the woody white core and thinly slice the leaves.
9. Keep them on the side.
10. Remove skillet from oven.

11. Transfer duck breast, fat side up to cutting board and let it rest.

12. Re-heat your skillet over medium heat.

13. Add unsalted butter, sage and cook for 3-4 minutes.

14. Cut duck into 6 equal slices.

15. Divide radicchio between 2 plates, top with slices of duck breast and drizzle browned butter and sage.

16. Enjoy!

Nutrition: Calories: 393; Fat: 33g; Carbohydrates: 2g; Protein: 22g

13. Generous Garlic Bread Stick

Preparation time: 15 minutes

Cooking time: 15 minutes

Servings: 8

Ingredients:

- ¼ cup almond butter, softened
- 1 teaspoon garlic powder
- 2 cups almond flour
- ½ tablespoon baking powder
- 1 tablespoon Psyllium husk powder
- ¼ teaspoon sunflower seeds
- 3 tablespoons almond butter, melted
- 1 egg
- ¼ cup boiling water

Directions:

1. Pre-heat your oven to 400 degrees F.
2. Line baking sheet with parchment paper and keep it on the side.
3. Beat almond butter with garlic powder and keep it on the side.
4. Add almond flour, baking powder, husk, sunflower seeds in a bowl and mix in almond butter and egg, mix well.

5. Pour boiling water in the mix and stir until you have a nice dough.

6. Divide the dough into 8 balls and roll into breadsticks.

7. Place on baking sheet and bake for 15 minutes.

8. Brush each stick with garlic almond butter and bake for 5 minutes more.

9. Serve and enjoy!

Nutrition: Total Carbs: 7g; Fiber: 2g; Protein: 7g; Fat: 24g

14. Cauliflower Bread Stick

Preparation time: 10 minutes

Cooking time: 48 minutes

Servings: 5

Ingredients:

- 1 cup cashew cheese/ kite ricotta cheese
- 1 tablespoon organic almond butter
- 1 whole egg
- ½ teaspoon Italian seasoning
- ¼ teaspoon red pepper flakes
- 1/8 teaspoon kosher sunflower seeds
- 2 cups cauliflower rice, cooked for 3 minutes in microwave
- 3 teaspoons garlic, minced
- Parmesan cheese, grated

Directions:

1. Pre-heat your oven to 350 degrees F.
2. Add almond butter in a small pan and melt over low heat
3. Add red pepper flakes, garlic to the almond butter and cook for 2-3 minutes.
4. Add garlic and almond butter mix to the bowl with cooked cauliflower and add the Italian seasoning.

5. Season with sunflower seeds and mix, refrigerate for 10 minutes.

6. Add cheese and eggs to the bowl and mix.

7. Place a layer of parchment paper at the bottom of a 9 x 9 baking dish and grease with cooking spray, add egg and mozzarella cheese mix to the cauliflower mix.

8. Add mix to the pan and smooth to a thin layer with the palms of your hand.

9. Bake for 30 minutes, take out from oven and top with few shakes of parmesan and mozzarella.

10. Cook for 8 minutes more.

11. Enjoy!

Nutrition: Total Carbs: 11.5g; Fiber: 2g; Protein: 10.7g; Fat: 20g

15. Bacon and Chicken Garlic Wrap

Preparation time: 15 minutes

Cooking time: 10 minutes

Servings: 4

Ingredients:

- 1 chicken fillet, cut into small cubes
- 8-9 thin slices bacon, cut to fit cubes
- 6 garlic cloves, minced

Directions:

1. Pre-heat your oven to 400 degrees F.
2. Line a baking tray with aluminum foil.
3. Add minced garlic to a bowl and rub each chicken piece with it.
4. Wrap a bacon piece around each garlic chicken bite.
5. Secure with toothpick.
6. Transfer bites to baking sheet, keeping a little bit of space between them.
7. Bake for about 15-20 minutes until crispy.
8. Serve and enjoy!

Nutrition: Calories: 260; Fat: 19g; Carbohydrates: 5g; Protein: 22g

MAINS

16. Tofu & Green Bean Stir-Fry

Preparation time: 15 minutes

Cooking time: 20 minutes

Servings: 4

Ingredients:

- 1 (14-ounce) package extra-firm tofu
- 2 tablespoons canola oil
- 1-pound green beans, chopped
- 2 carrots, peeled and thinly sliced
- ½ cup Stir-Fry Sauce or store-bought lower-sodium stir-fry sauce
- 2 cups Fluffy Brown Rice
- 2 scallions, thinly sliced
- 2 tablespoons sesame seeds

Directions:

1. Put the tofu on your plate lined with a kitchen towel, put separate kitchen towel over the tofu, and place a heavy pot on top, changing towels every time they become soaked. Let sit within 15 minutes to remove the moisture. Cut the tofu into 1-inch cubes.

2. Heat the canola oil in a large wok or skillet to medium-high heat. Add the tofu cubes and cook, flipping every 1 to 2 minutes, so all sides become browned. Remove from the skillet and place the green beans and carrots in the hot oil. Stir-fry for 4 to 5 minutes, occasionally tossing, until crisp and slightly tender.

3. While the vegetables are cooking, prepare the Stir-Fry Sauce (if using homemade). Place the tofu back in the skillet. Put the sauce over the tofu and vegetables and let simmer for 2 to 3 minutes. Serve over rice, then top with scallions and sesame seeds.

Nutrition: Calories: 380, Fat: 15g, Sodium: 440mg, Potassium: 454mg, Carbohydrate: 45g, Protein: 16g

17. <u>Peanut Vegetable Pad Thai</u>

Preparation time: 15 minutes

Cooking time: 20 minutes

Servings: 6

Ingredients:

- 8 ounces brown rice noodles
- 1/3 cup natural peanut butter
- 3 tablespoons unsalted vegetable broth
- 1 tablespoon low-sodium soy sauce
- 2 tablespoons of rice wine vinegar
- 1 tablespoon honey
- 2 teaspoons sesame oil
- 1 teaspoon sriracha (optional)
- 1 tablespoon canola oil
- 1 red bell pepper, thinly sliced
- 1 zucchini, cut into matchsticks
- 2 large carrots, cut into matchsticks
- 3 large eggs, beaten
- ¾ teaspoon kosher or sea salt
- ½ cup unsalted peanuts, chopped
- ½ cup cilantro leaves, chopped

Directions:

1. Boil a large pot of water. Cook the rice noodles as stated in package directions. Mix the peanut butter, vegetable broth, soy sauce, rice wine vinegar, honey, sesame oil, and sriracha in a bowl. Set aside.

2. Warm-up canola oil over medium heat in a large nonstick skillet. Add the red bell pepper, zucchini, and carrots, and sauté for 2 to 3 minutes, until slightly soft. Stir in the eggs and fold with a spatula until scrambled. Add the cooked rice noodles, sauce, and salt. Toss to combine. Spoon into bowls and evenly top with the peanuts and cilantro.

Nutrition: Calories: 393, Fat: 19g, Sodium: 561mg, Carbohydrate: 45g, Protein: 13g

18. Spicy Tofu Burrito Bowls with Cilantro Avocado Sauce

Preparation time: 15 minutes

Cooking time: 15 minutes

Servings: 4

Ingredients:

- For the sauce:
- ¼ cup plain nonfat Greek yogurt
- ½ cup fresh cilantro leaves
- ½ ripe avocado, peeled
- Zest and juice of 1 lime
- 2 garlic cloves, peeled
- ¼ teaspoon kosher or sea salt
- 2 tablespoons water
- For the burrito bowls:
- 1 (14-ounce) package extra-firm tofu
- 1 tablespoon canola oil
- 1 yellow or orange bell pepper, diced
- 2 tablespoons Taco Seasoning
- ¼ teaspoon kosher or sea salt
- 2 cups Fluffy Brown Rice
- 1 (15-ounce) can black beans, drained

Directions:

1. Place all the sauce ingredients in the bowl of a food processor or blender and purée until smooth. Taste and adjust the seasoning, if necessary. Refrigerate until ready for use.

2. Put the tofu on your plate lined with a kitchen towel. Put another kitchen towel over the tofu and place a heavy pot on top, changing towels if they become soaked. Let it stand within 15 minutes to remove the moisture. Cut the tofu into 1-inch cubes.

3. Warm-up canola oil in a large skillet over medium heat. Add the tofu and bell pepper and sauté, breaking up the tofu into smaller pieces for 4 to 5 minutes. Stir in the taco seasoning, salt, and ¼ cup of water. Evenly divide the rice and black beans among 4 bowls. Top with the tofu/bell pepper mixture and top with the cilantro avocado sauce.

Nutrition: Calories: 383, Fat: 13g, Sodium: 438mg, Carbohydrate: 48g, Protein: 21g

19. **Sweet Potato Cakes with Classic Guacamole**

Preparation time: 15 minutes

Cooking time: 20 minutes

Servings: 4

Ingredients:

- For the guacamole:
- 2 ripe avocados, peeled and pitted
- ½ jalapeño, seeded and finely minced
- ¼ red onion, peeled and finely diced
- ¼ cup fresh cilantro leaves, chopped
- Zest and juice of 1 lime
- ¼ teaspoon kosher or sea salt
- For the cakes:
- 3 sweet potatoes, cooked and peeled
- ½ cup cooked black beans
- 1 large egg
- ½ cup panko bread crumbs
- 1 teaspoon ground cumin
- 1 teaspoon chili powder
- ½ teaspoon kosher or sea salt
- ¼ teaspoon ground black pepper
- 2 tablespoons canola oil

Directions:

1. Mash the avocado, then stir in the jalapeño, red onion, cilantro, lime zest and juice, and salt in a bowl. Taste and adjust the seasoning, if necessary.

2. Put the cooked sweet potatoes plus black beans in a bowl and mash until a paste form. Stir in the egg, bread crumbs, cumin, chili powder, salt, and black pepper until combined.

3. Warm-up canola oil in a large skillet at medium heat. Form the sweet potato mixture into 4 patties, place them in the hot skillet, and cook within 3 to 4 minutes per side, until browned and crispy. Serve the sweet potato cakes with guacamole on top.

Nutrition: Calories: 369, Fat: 22g, Sodium: 521mg, Carbohydrate: 38g, Protein: 8g

20. <u>Chickpea Cauliflower Tikka Masala</u>

Preparation time: 15 minutes

Cooking time: 40 minutes

Servings: 6

Ingredients:

- 2 tablespoons olive oil
- 1 yellow onion, peeled and diced
- 4 garlic cloves, peeled and minced
- 1-inch piece fresh ginger, peeled and minced
- 2 tablespoons Garam Masala
- 1 teaspoon kosher or sea salt
- ½ teaspoon ground black pepper
- ¼ teaspoon ground cayenne pepper
- ½ small head cauliflower, small florets
- 2 (15-ounce) cans no-salt-added chickpeas, rinsed and drained
- 1 (15-ounce) can no-salt-added petite diced tomatoes, drained
- 1½ cups unsalted vegetable broth
- ½ (15-ounce) can coconut milk
- Zest and juice of 1 lime
- ½ cup fresh cilantro leaves, chopped, divided
- 1½ cups cooked Fluffy Brown Rice, divided

Directions:

1. Warm-up olive oil over medium heat, then put the onion and sauté within 4 to 5 minutes in a large Dutch oven or stockpot. Stir in the garlic, ginger, garam masala, salt, black pepper, and cayenne pepper and toast for 30 to 60 seconds, until fragrant.

2. Stir in the cauliflower florets, chickpeas, diced tomatoes, and vegetable broth and increase to medium-high. Simmer within 15 minutes, until the cauliflower is fork-tender.

3. Remove, then stir in the coconut milk, lime juice, lime zest, and half of the cilantro. Taste and adjust the seasoning, if necessary. Serve over the rice and the remaining chopped cilantro.

Nutrition: Calories: 323, Fat: 12g, Sodium: 444mg, Carbohydrate: 44g, Protein: 11g

SIDES & APPETIZERS

21. Easy Carrots Mix

Preparation time: 10 minutes

Cooking time: 40 minutes

Servings: 6

Ingredients:

- 15 carrots, halved lengthwise
- 2 tablespoons coconut sugar
- ¼ cup olive oil
- ½ teaspoon rosemary, dried
- ½ teaspoon garlic powder
- A pinch of black pepper

Directions:

1. In a bowl, combine the carrots with the sugar, oil, rosemary, garlic powder, and black pepper, toss well, spread on a lined baking sheet, introduce in the oven and bake at 400 degrees F for 40 minutes. Serve.

Nutrition: Calories: 60; Carbs: 9g; Fat: 0g; Protein: 2g; Sodium: 0 mg

22. Tasty Grilled Asparagus

Preparation time: 10 minutes

Cooking time: 6 minutes

Servings: 4

Ingredients:

- 2 pounds asparagus, trimmed
- 2 tablespoons olive oil
- A pinch of salt and black pepper

Directions:

1. In a bowl, combine the asparagus with salt, pepper, and oil and toss well. Place the asparagus on a preheated grill over medium-high heat, cook for 3 minutes on each side, then serve.

Nutrition: Calories: 50; Carbs: 8g; Fat: 1g; Protein: 5g; Sodium: 420 mg

23. Roasted Carrots

Preparation time: 10 minutes

Cooking time: 30 minutes

Servings: 4

Ingredients:

- 2 pounds carrots, quartered
- A pinch of black pepper
- 3 tablespoons olive oil
- 2 tablespoons parsley, chopped

Directions:

1. Arrange the carrots on a lined baking sheet, add black pepper and oil, toss, introduce in the oven, and cook within 30 minutes at 400 degrees F. Add parsley, toss, divide between plates and serve as a side dish.

Nutrition: Calories: 89; Carbs: 10g; Fat: 6g; Protein: 1g; Sodium: 0 mg

24. Oven Roasted Asparagus

Preparation time: 10 minutes

Cooking time: 25 minutes

Servings: 4

Ingredients:

- 2 pounds asparagus spears, trimmed
- 3 tablespoons olive oil
- A pinch of black pepper
- 2 teaspoons sweet paprika
- 1 teaspoon sesame seeds

Directions:

1. Arrange the asparagus on a lined baking sheet, add oil, black pepper, and paprika, toss, introduce in the oven and bake within 25 minutes at 400 degrees F. Divide the asparagus between plates, sprinkle sesame seeds on top, and serve as a side dish.

Nutrition: Calories: 45; Carbs: 5g; Fat: 2g; Protein: 2g; Sodium: 0 mg

25. **Baked Potato with Thyme**

Preparation time: 10 minutes

Cooking time: 1 hour and 15 minutes

Servings: 8

Ingredients:

- 6 potatoes, peeled and sliced
- 2 garlic cloves, minced
- 2 tablespoons olive oil
- 1 and ½ cups of coconut cream
- ¼ cup of coconut milk
- 1 tablespoon thyme, chopped
- ¼ teaspoon nutmeg, ground
- A pinch of red pepper flakes
- 1 and ½ cups low-fat cheddar, shredded
- ½ cup low-fat parmesan, grated

Directions:

1. Heat-up a pan with the oil over medium heat, add garlic, stir and cook for 1 minute. Add coconut cream, coconut milk, thyme, nutmeg, and pepper flakes, stir, bring to a simmer, adjust to low and cook within 10 minutes.

2. Put one-third of the potatoes in a baking dish, add 1/3 of the cream, repeat the process with the remaining potatoes and the cream, sprinkle the cheddar on top,

cover with tin foil, introduce in the oven and cook at 375 degrees F for 45 minutes. Uncover the dish, sprinkle the parmesan, bake everything for 20 minutes, divide between plates, and serve as a side dish.

Nutrition: Calories: 132; Carbs: 21g; Fat: 4g; Protein: 2g; Sodium: 56 mg

SEAFOOD

26. Roasted Lemon Swordfish

Preparation time: 10 minutes

Cooking Time: 70-80 minutes

Servings: 4

Ingredients:

- ¼ cup parsley, chopped
- ½ teaspoon garlic, chopped
- ½ teaspoon canola oil
- 4 swordfish fillets, 6 ounces each
- ¼ teaspoon sunflower seeds
- tablespoon sugar
- lemons, quartered and seeds removed

Directions:

1. Preheat your oven to 375 degrees F.
2. Take a small-sized bowl and add sugar, sunflower seeds, lemon wedges.
3. Toss well to coat them.
4. Take a shallow baking dish and add lemons, cover with aluminum foil.
5. Roast for about 60 minutes until lemons are tender and browned (Slightly).

6. Heat your grill and place the rack about 4 inches away from the source of heat.

7. Take a baking pan and coat it with cooking spray.

8. Transfer fish fillets to the pan and brush with oil on top spread garlic on top.

9. Grill for about 5 minutes each side until fillet turns opaque.

10. Transfer fish to a serving platter, squeeze roasted lemon on top.

11. Sprinkle parsley serve with a lemon wedge on the side.

12. Enjoy!

Nutrition: Calories: 280; Fat: 12g; Net Carbohydrates: 4g; Protein: 34g

27. **Especial Glazed Salmon**

Preparation time: 45 minutes

Cooking Time: 10 minutes

Serving: 4

Ingredients:

- 4 pieces salmon fillets, 5 ounces each
- 4 tablespoons coconut aminos
- 4 teaspoon olive oil
- 2 teaspoons ginger, minced
- 4 teaspoons garlic, minced
- 2 tablespoons sugar-free ketchup
- 4 tablespoons dry white wine
- 2 tablespoons red boat fish sauce, low sodium

Directions:

1. Take a bowl and mix in coconut aminos, garlic, ginger, fish sauce and mix.
2. Add salmon and let it marinate for 15-20 minutes.
3. Take a skillet/pan and place it over medium heat.
4. Add oil and let it heat up.
5. Add salmon fillets and cook on high heat for 3-4 minutes per side.
6. Remove dish once crispy.
7. Add sauce and wine.

8. Simmer for 5 minutes on low heat.

9. Return salmon to the glaze and flip until both sides are glazed.

10. Serve and enjoy!

Nutrition: Calories: 372; Fat: 24g; Carbohydrates: 3g; Protein: 35g

28. Generous Stuffed Salmon Avocado

Preparation time: 10 minutes

Cooking Time: 30 minutes

Serving: 2

Ingredients:

- ripe organic avocado
- ounces wild caught smoked salmon
- ounce cashew cheese
- tablespoons extra virgin olive oil
- Sunflower seeds as needed

Directions:

1. Cut avocado in half and deseed.
2. Add the rest of the ingredients to a food processor and process until coarsely chopped.
3. Place mixture into avocado.
4. Serve and enjoy!

Nutrition: Calories: 525; Fat: 48g; Carbohydrates: 4g; Protein: 19g

29. Spanish Mussels

Preparation time: 10 minutes

Cooking Time: 23 minutes

Serving: 4

Ingredients:

- 3 tablespoons olive oil
- 2 pounds mussels, scrubbed
- Pepper to taste
- 3 cups canned tomatoes, crushed
- shallot, chopped
- garlic cloves, minced
- cups low sodium vegetable stock
- 1/3 cup cilantro, chopped

Directions:

1. Take a pan and place it over medium-high heat, add shallot and stir-cook for 3 minutes.
2. Add garlic, stock, tomatoes, pepper, stir and reduce heat, simmer for 10 minutes.
3. Add mussels, cilantro, and toss.
4. Cover and cook for 10 minutes more.
5. Serve and enjoy!

Nutrition: Calories: 210; Fat: 2g; Carbohydrates: 5g; Protein: 8g

30. Tilapia Broccoli Platter

Preparation time: 4 minutes

Cooking Time: 14 minutes

Serving: 2

Ingredients:

- 6 ounce tilapia, frozen
- tablespoon almond butter
- tablespoon garlic, minced
- 1 teaspoon lemon pepper seasoning
- 1 cup broccoli florets, fresh

Directions:

1. Preheat your oven to 350 degrees F.
2. Add fish in aluminum foil packets.
3. Arrange broccoli around fish.
4. Sprinkle lemon pepper on top.
5. Close the packets and seal.
6. Bake for 14 minutes.
7. Take a bowl and add garlic and almond butter, mix well and keep the mixture on the side.
8. Remove the packet from oven and transfer to platter.
9. Place almond butter on top of the fish and broccoli, serve and enjoy!

Nutrition: Calories: 362; Fat: 25g; Carbohydrates: 2g; Protein: 29g

31. Olive Capers Chicken

Preparation time: 15 minutes

Cooking time: 16 minutes

Servings: 4

Ingredients:

- 2 lbs. chicken
- 1/3 cup chicken stock
- oz. Capers
- 6 oz. olives
- 1/4 cup fresh basil
- 1 tbsp. olive oil
- 1 tsp. oregano
- 2 garlic cloves, minced
- 2 tbsp. red wine vinegar
- 1/8 tsp. pepper
- 1/4 tsp. salt

Directions:

1. Put olive oil in your instant pot and set the pot on sauté mode. Add chicken to the pot and sauté for 3-4 minutes. Add remaining ingredients and stir well. Seal

pot with the lid and select manual and set timer for 12 minutes. Serve and enjoy.

Nutrition: Calories: 433 Fat: 15.2g Protein: 66.9g Carbs: 4.8g Sodium 244 mg

32. Chicken with Mushrooms

Preparation time: 15 minutes

Cooking time: 6 hours & 10 minutes

Servings: 2

Ingredients:

- 2 chicken breasts, skinless and boneless
- 1 cup mushrooms, sliced
- 1 onion, sliced
- 1 cup chicken stock
- 1/2 tsp. thyme, dried
- Pepper
- Salt

Directions:

1. Add all ingredients to the slow cooker. Cook on low within 6 hours. Serve and enjoy.

Nutrition: Calories: 313 Fat: 11.3g Protein: 44.3g Carbs: 6.9g Sodium 541 mg

33. Baked Chicken

Preparation time: 15 minutes

Cooking time: 35 minutes

Servings: 4

Ingredients:

- 2 lbs. chicken tenders
- 1 large zucchini
- 1 cup grape tomatoes
- 2 tbsp. olive oil
- 3 dill sprigs
- For topping:
- 2 tbsp. feta cheese, crumbled
- 1 tbsp. olive oil
- 1 tbsp. fresh lemon juice
- 1 tbsp. fresh dill, chopped

Directions:

1. Warm oven to 200 C/ 400 F. Drizzle the olive oil on a baking tray, then place chicken, zucchini, dill, and tomatoes on the tray. Season with salt. Bake chicken within 30 minutes.

2. Meanwhile, in a small bowl, stir all topping ingredients. Place chicken on the serving tray, then top with veggies and discard dill sprigs. Sprinkle topping

mixture on top of chicken and vegetables. Serve and enjoy.

Nutrition: Calories: 557 Fat: 28.6g Protein: 67.9g Carbs: 5.2g Sodium 760 mg

34. Garlic Pepper Chicken

Preparation time: 15 minutes

Cooking time: 21 minutes

Servings: 2

Ingredients:

- 2 chicken breasts, cut into strips
- 2 bell peppers, cut into strips
- 5 garlic cloves, chopped
- 3 tbsp. water
- 2 tbsp. olive oil
- 1 tbsp. paprika
- 2 tsp. black pepper
- 1/2 tsp. salt

Directions:

1. Warm-up olive oil in a large saucepan over medium heat. Add garlic and sauté for 2-3 minutes. Add peppers and cook for 3 minutes. Add chicken and spices and stir to coat. Add water and stir well. Bring to boil. Cover and simmer for 10-15 minutes. Serve and enjoy.

Nutrition: Calories: 462 Fat: 25.7g Protein: 44.7g Carbs: 14.8g Sodium 720 mg

35. Mustard Chicken Tenders

Preparation time: 15 minutes

Cooking time: 20 minutes

Servings: 4

Ingredients:

- 1 lb. chicken tenders
- 2 tbsp. fresh tarragon, chopped
- 1/2 cup whole grain mustard
- 1/2 tsp. paprika
- 1 garlic clove, minced
- 1/2 oz. fresh lemon juice
- 1/2 tsp. pepper
- 1/4 tsp. kosher salt

Directions:

1. Warm oven to 425 F. Add all ingredients except chicken to the large bowl and mix well. Put the chicken in the bowl, then stir until well coated. Place chicken on a baking dish and cover. Bake within 15-20 minutes. Serve and enjoy.

Nutrition: Calories: 242 Fat: 9.5g Protein: 33.2g Carbs: 3.1g Sodium 240 mg

MEAT

36. Pork, Water Chestnuts and Cabbage Salad

Preparation time: 10 minutes

Cooking time: 0 minutes

Servings: 10

Ingredients:

- 1 green cabbage head, shredded
- 1 and ½ cups brown rice, already cooked
- 2 cups pork roast, already cooked and shredded
- 10 ounces peas
- 8 ounces water chestnuts, drained and sliced
- ½ cup low-fat sour cream
- ½ cup avocado mayonnaise
- A pinch of black pepper

Directions:

1. In a bowl, combine the cabbage with the rice, shredded meat, peas, chestnuts, sour cream, mayo and black pepper, toss and serve cold.
2. Enjoy!

Nutrition: Calories 310, Fat 5, Fiber 4, Carbs 11, Protein 17

37. Pork and Zucchini Stew

Preparation time: 10 minutes

Cooking time: 1 hour

Servings: 4

Ingredients:

- 1 pound ground pork, cubed
- Black pepper to the taste
- ¼ teaspoon sweet paprika
- 1 tablespoon olive oil
- 1 and ½ cups low-sodium veggie stock
- 3 cups zucchinis, cubed
- 1 yellow onion, chopped
- ½ cup low-sodium tomato sauce
- 1 tablespoon parsley, chopped

Directions:

1. Heat up a pot with the oil over medium-high heat, add the pork, black pepper and paprika, stir and brown for 5 minutes.

2. Add stock, onion and tomato sauce, toss, bring to a simmer, reduce heat to medium and cook for 40 minutes.

3. Add the zucchinis and the parsley, toss, cook for 15 minutes more, divide into bowls and serve.

4. Enjoy!

Nutrition: Calories 270, Fat 7, Fiber 9, Carbs 12, Protein 17

38. Pork Roast, Leeks and Carrots

Preparation time: 10 minutes

Cooking time: 1 hour and 10 minutes

Servings: 4

Ingredients:

- 2 pounds pork roast, trimmed
- 4 carrots, chopped
- 4 leeks, chopped
- 1 teaspoon black peppercorns
- 2 yellow onions, cut into wedges
- 1 tablespoon parsley, chopped
- 1 cup low-sodium veggie stock
- 1 teaspoon mustard
- Black pepper to the taste

Directions:

1. Put the pork in a roasting pan, add carrots, leeks, peppercorns, onions, stock, mustard and black pepper, toss, cover the pan and bake in the oven at 375 degrees F for 1 hour and 10 minutes.

2. Slice the meat, divide it between plates, sprinkle parsley on top and serve with the carrots and leeks mix on the side.

3. Enjoy!

Nutrition: Calories 260, Fat 5, Fiber 7, Carbs 12, Protein 20

39. Easy Veal Chops

Preparation time: 10 minutes

Cooking time: 20 minutes

Servings: 4

Ingredients:

- 3 tablespoons whole wheat flour
- Black pepper to the taste
- 2 eggs
- 1 tablespoon milk
- 1 and ½ cups whole wheat breadcrumbs
- Zest of 1 lemon, grated
- 4 veal rib chops
- 3 tablespoons olive oil

Directions:

1. Put whole wheat flour in a bowl.
2. In another bowl, mix eggs with milk and whisk
3. In a third bowl, mix the breadcrumbs with lemon zest.
4. Season veal chops with black pepper, dredge them in flour, dip in the egg mix and then in breadcrumbs.
5. Heat up a pan with the oil over medium-high heat, add veal chops, cook for 2 minutes on each side and transfer to a baking sheet, introduce them in the oven at 350 degrees F, bake for 15 minutes, divide between plates and serve with a side salad.

6. Enjoy!

Nutrition: Calories 270, Fat 6, Fiber 7, Carbs 10, Protein 16

40. **Pork with Apple Sauce**

Preparation time: 10 minutes

Cooking time: 1 hour and 30 minutes

Servings: 6

Ingredients:

- 1 tablespoon lemon juice
- 2 cups low-sodium veggie stock
- 17 ounces apples, cored and cut into wedges
- 2 pounds pork belly, trimmed and scored
- 1 teaspoons sweet paprika
- Black pepper to the taste
- A drizzle of olive oil

Directions:

1. In your blender, mix the stock with apples and lemon juice and pulse very well.

2. Put pork belly in a roasting pan, add apple sauce, also add the oil, paprika and black pepper, toss well, introduce in the oven and bake at 380 degrees F for 1 hour and 30 minutes.

3. Slice the pork belly, divide it between plates, drizzle the sauce all over and serve.

4. Enjoy!

Nutrition: Calories 356, Fat 14, Fiber 4, Carbs 10, Protein 27

VEGETABLES

41. Southwestern Bean-And-Pepper Salad

Preparation time: 6 minutes

Cooking time: 0 minutes

Servings: 4

Ingredients:

- 1 can pinto beans, drained
- 2 bell peppers, cored and chopped
- 1 cup corn kernels
- Salt
- Freshly ground black pepper
- Juice of 2 limes
- 1 tablespoon olive oil
- 1 avocado, chopped

Directions:

1. Mix beans, peppers, corn, salt, plus pepper in a large bowl. Press fresh lime juice, then mix in olive oil. Let the salad stand in the fridge within 30 minutes. Add avocado just before serving.

Nutrition: Calories: 245; Fat: 11g; Sodium: 97mg; Carbohydrate: 32g; Protein: 8g

42. Cauliflower Mashed Potatoes

Preparation time: 10 minutes

Cooking time: 10 minutes

Servings: 4

Ingredients:

- 16 cups water (enough to cover cauliflower)
- 1 head cauliflower (about 3 pounds), trimmed and cut into florets
- 4 garlic cloves
- 1 tablespoon olive oil
- ¼ teaspoon salt
- 1/8 teaspoon freshly ground black pepper
- 2 teaspoons dried parsley

Directions:

1. Boil a large pot of water, then the cauliflower and garlic. Cook within 10 minutes, then strain. Move it back to the hot pan, and let it stand within 2 to 3 minutes with the lid on.

2. Put the cauliflower plus garlic in a food processor or blender. Add the olive oil, salt, pepper, and purée until smooth. Taste and adjust the salt and pepper.

3. Remove, then put the parsley, and mix until combined. Garnish with additional olive oil, if desired. Serve immediately.

Nutrition: Calories: 87g; Fat: 4g; Sodium: 210mg; Carbohydrate: 12g; Protein: 4g

43. Roasted Brussels sprouts

Preparation time: 5 minutes

Cooking time: 20 minutes

Servings: 4

Ingredients:

- 1½ pounds Brussels sprouts, trimmed and halved
- 2 tablespoons olive oil
- ¼ teaspoon salt
- ½ teaspoon freshly ground black pepper

Directions:

1. Preheat the oven to 400°f. Combine the Brussels sprouts and olive oil in a large mixing bowl and toss until they are evenly coated.

2. Turn the Brussels sprouts out onto a large baking sheet and flip them over, so they are cut-side down with the flat part touching the baking sheet. Sprinkle with salt and pepper.

3. Bake within 20 to 30 minutes or until the Brussels sprouts are lightly charred and crisp on the outside and toasted on the bottom. The outer leaves will be extra dark, too. Serve immediately.

Nutrition: Calories: 134; Fat: 8g; Sodium: 189mg; Carbohydrate: 15g; Protein: 6g

44. Broccoli with Garlic and Lemon

Preparation time: 2 minutes

Cooking time: 4 minutes

Servings: 4

Ingredients:

- 1 cup of water
- 4 cups broccoli florets
- 1 teaspoon olive oil
- 1 tablespoon minced garlic
- 1 teaspoon lemon zest
- Salt
- Freshly ground black pepper

Directions:

1. Put the broccoli in the boiling water in a small saucepan and cook within 2 to 3 minutes. The broccoli should retain its bright-green color. Drain the water from the broccoli.

2. Put the olive oil in a small sauté pan over medium-high heat. Add the garlic and sauté for 30 seconds. Put the broccoli, lemon zest, salt, plus pepper. Combine well and serve.

Nutrition: Calories: 38g; Fat: 1g; Sodium: 24mg; Carbohydrate: 5g; Protein: 3g

45. Brown Rice Pilaf

Preparation time: 5 minutes

Cooking time: 10 minutes

Servings: 4

Ingredients:

- 1 cup low-sodium vegetable broth
- ½ tablespoon olive oil
- 1 clove garlic, minced
- 1 scallion, thinly sliced
- 1 tablespoon minced onion flakes
- 1 cup instant brown rice
- 1/8 teaspoon freshly ground black pepper

Directions:

1. Mix the vegetable broth, olive oil, garlic, scallion, and minced onion flakes in a saucepan and boil. Put rice, then boil it again, adjust the heat and simmer within 10 minutes. Remove and let stand within 5 minutes. Fluff with a fork and season with black pepper.

Nutrition: Calories: 100g; Fat: 2g; Sodium: 35mg; Carbohydrate: 19g; Protein: 2g

SNACK AND DESSERTS

46. Summer Jam

Preparation time: 10 minutes

Cooking time: 3 hours

Servings: 6

Ingredients:

- 2 cups coconut sugar
- 4 cups cherries, pitted
- 2 tablespoons lemon juice
- 3 tablespoons gelatin

Directions:

1. In your slow cooker, mix lemon juice with gelatin, cherries and coconut sugar, stir, cover, cook on High for 3 hours, divide into bowls and serve cold.

Nutrition: Calories 171, Fat 0.1g, Cholesterol 0mg, Sodium 41mg, Carbohydrate 37.2g, Fiber 0.7g, Sugars 0.1g, Protein 3.8g, Potassium 122mg

47. Cinnamon Pudding

Preparation time: 10 minutes

Cooking time: 5 hours

Servings: 4

Ingredients:

- 2 cups white rice
- 1 cup coconut sugar
- 2 cinnamon sticks
- **6** and ½ cups water
- ½ cup coconut, shredded

Directions:

1. In your slow cooker, mix water with the rice, sugar, cinnamon and coconut, stir, cover, cook on High for 5 hours, discard cinnamon, divide pudding into bowls and serve warm.

Nutrition: Calories 400, Fat 4g, Cholesterol 0mg, Sodium 28mg, Carbohydrate 81.2g, Fiber 2.7g, Sugars 0.8g, Protein 7.2g, Potassium 151mg

48. Orange Compote

Preparation time: 10 minutes

Cooking time: 2 hours and 30 minutes

Servings: 4

Ingredients:

- ½ pound oranges, peeled and cut into segments
- ½ pound plums, pitted and halved
- 1 cup orange juice
- 3 tablespoons coconut sugar
- ½ cup water

Directions:

1. In the slow cooker, combine the oranges with the plums, orange juice and the other ingredients, put the lid on and cook on High for 2 hours and 30 minutes.
2. Stir, divide into bowls and serve cold.

Nutrition: Calories 130, Fat 0.2g, Cholesterol 0mg, Sodium 31mg, Carbohydrate 28.4g, Fiber 1.6g, Sugars 11.4g, Protein 1.8g, Potassium 240mg

49. Chocolate Bars

Preparation time: 10 minutes

Cooking time: 2 hours and 30 minutes

Servings: 12

Ingredients:

- 1 cup coconut sugar
- ½ cup dark chocolate chips
- 1 egg white
- ¼ cup coconut oil, melted
- ½ teaspoon vanilla extract
- 1 teaspoon baking powder
- 1 and ½ cups almond meal

Directions:

1. In a bowl, mix the oil with sugar, vanilla extract, egg white, baking powder and almond flour and whisk well
2. Fold in chocolate chips and stir gently.
3. Line your slow cooker with parchment paper, grease it, add cookie mix, press on the bottom, cover and cook on low for 2 hours and 30 minutes.
4. Take cookie sheet out of the slow cooker, cut into medium bars and serve.

Nutrition: Calories 141, Fat 11.8g, Cholesterol 0mg, Sodium 7mg, Carbohydrate 7.7g, Fiber 1.5g, Sugars 3.2g, Protein 3.2g, Potassium 134mg

50. Lemon Zest Pudding

Preparation time: 10 minutes

Cooking time: 5 hours

Servings: 4

Ingredients:

- 1 cup pineapple juice, natural
- Cooking spray
- 1 teaspoon baking powder
- 1 cup coconut flour
- 3 tablespoons avocado oil
- 3 tablespoons stevia
- ½ cup pineapple, chopped
- ½ cup lemon zest, grated
- ½ cup coconut milk
- ½ cup pecans, chopped

Directions:

1. Spray your slow cooker with cooking spray.
2. In a bowl, mix flour with stevia, baking powder, oil, milk, pecans, pineapple, lemon zest and pineapple juice, stir well, pour into your slow cooker greased with cooking spray, cover and cook on Low for 5 hours.
3. Divide into bowls and serve.

Nutrition: Calories 431, Fat 29.7g, Cholesterol 0mg, Sodium 8mg, Carbohydrate 47.1g, Fiber 17g, Sugars 10.9g, Protein 8.1g, Potassium 482mg

CPSIA information can be obtained
at www.ICGtesting.com
Printed in the USA
BVHW091017300421
605944BV00027B/964